■ 'A moderate intake of sugar-rich foods can provide for a palatable and nutritious diet.'

■ 'There is no evidence of a direct involvement of sucrose, other sugars and starch in the etiology of lifestyle-related diseases.'

—United Nations FAO/WHO
Expert Consultation on Carbohydrates, 1998

the Pocket Guide to the
glucose
revolution
and sugar and energy

ASSOC. PROFESSOR JENNIE BRAND-MILLER • KAYE FOSTER-POWELL
DR ANTHONY LEEDS

coronet

First published in Australia in 1999 by
Hodder Headline Australia Pty Limited

First published in Great Britain in 2002 by Hodder and Stoughton
A division of Hodder Headline

This United Kingdom edition is published by arrangement with
Hodder Headline Australia Pty Limited
A Coronet paperback

10 9 8 7 6 5 4 3 2 1

A CIP catalogue record for this title is available from the British Library

0 340 77057 0

Typeset in Minion and Gill Sans by
Phoenix Typesetting, Ilkley, West Yorkshire

Printed and bound in Great Britain by Omnia Books Ltd, Glasgow

Hodder and Stoughton
A division of Hodder Headline
338 Euston Road
London NW1 3BH

CONTENTS

INTRODUCTION

Many people today are convinced that sugar is a real 'no-no' – one of the evils of modern diets and responsible (virtually on its own!) for a multitude of human diseases. Others are not quite so negative, but still regard sugar as one of those things people can easily do without – because it's simply not necessary and you benefit by avoiding it.

These messages are what many doctors, dentists, nutritionists and health authorities have preached for many years – and some still hold fast to these opinions, despite the scientific evidence we now have. Their negative views of sugar stem from studies in the 1960s and 1970s that associated sugar with 'empty calories', rapid weight gain (in rats!) and dental decay. Nutrition science and public health have progressed markedly since then, but unfortunately some of the mud still sticks.

For the past twenty years, sugar has been the subject of close scientific scrutiny worldwide and the evidence from hundreds of studies clearly indicates that sugar is not the villain it was once thought to be. In the opinion of the world's leading nutrition authorities including the World Health Organisation and the Food and Agriculture Organisation of the United Nations, moderate intake of sugar-rich foods can provide for a palatable and nutritious diet.

If we look at the recent scientific evidence objectively,

the findings suggest that avoiding sugar may do you more harm than good. There are undesirable aspects of diets that are low in sugars. The vast array of sugar-free and 'no added sugar' foods on supermarket shelves has not solved the problem of overweight and obesity. In fact, it could be said that they have exacerbated the problem.

In this book we take a look at the scientifically proven breakthroughs about sugar and energy; dispel some common myths; reveal why it's high time to get rid of the guilt; and tell you what you really need to know about sugar, your health and blood sugar control, weight loss, dental decay and behaviour and mental performance.

Our intention is not to encourage an excessive amount of sugar. Excess of anything is not a good idea! We want you to feel that your normal instincts will guide you to eat a moderate quantity of sugar – the amount that is eaten by the average consumer – about 60 grams of refined sugar per day for an adult. This little book tells you what this means in real diets with sample menus for adults, children and people with diabetes.

WHAT WE MEAN BY ENERGY

In a nutritional sense, 'energy' equals the kilocalories (or kilojoules) that become available when a food is digested and metabolised within the body. The energy content of a food provides a measure of that food's capacity to provide our fuel requirements. Some foods provide more energy than others. High fat foods have the greatest energy content (fat has 9 kcal/g), high sugar foods have less than half the energy content of high fat foods (sugar has 4 kcal/g). Their energy content is similar to that of high protein foods (protein has 4 kcal/g).

WHAT IS SUGAR'S ROLE IN OUR DIET?

Sugar plays a unique role in our diet. No other nutrient satisfies our natural (instinctive) desire for sweetness. There are also some healthy reasons to include a moderate amount of sugar in your diet. It will help you

- maintain an ideal weight
- reduce your intake of saturated fat
- maximise your micronutrient intake

Sugar also has several functional roles in our food supply including preservative, textural and flavour-modifying qualities. When we take sugar out of foods we have to add other ingredients to do the job – intense sweeteners to replace the sweetness, fat or maltodextrins to replace the bulk and texture, preservatives to replace the anti-microbial qualities of sugar.

WHAT IS A MODERATE INTAKE?

Moderate intake of sugar means about 50–60 grams of refined sugar a day. This is the average amount of sugar eaten by people in industrialised countries like Britain. It includes all sources of refined sugar – that in soft drinks, confectionery, cakes and biscuits as well as that which we add ourselves to tea, coffee and breakfast cereals.

IS OUR LIKING FOR SWEETNESS INSTINCTIVE?

Sugars in fruit and honey have provided carbohydrate energy in human diets for millions of years – ever since primates began involving on a steady diet of fruit and berries in the rainforests of Africa 50 million years ago.

The appreciation of the sensation of sweetness runs deep in the human psyche. In literature and mythology, sweetness is linked with pleasure and goodness and in everyday language we use terms associated with sweetness to describe the things we love (sweetie pie, honeymoon). Our first food, breast milk, is sweet – in fact the sweetest of all mammalian milks. Infants smile when you offer them a sweet solution and cry if you give them something sour or bitter.

Sweetness is not a learned taste: everyone could be said to be born with a 'sweet tooth'. The reason for this preference is not known but may be related to our brain's dependence on glucose as its sole source of fuel. Perhaps those early human beings who were most able to detect sweetness were those most likely to survive. In fact, modern day monkeys that seek out fruit and berries have larger brains than those that survive on the leaves close at hand.

Our hunter-gatherer ancestors relished honey and other sources of concentrated sugars such as maple syrup, dried fruit and honey ants. Wild honey was so highly prized that we went to great lengths to obtain it.

- Australian Aborigines would attach a tiny feather to a bee and follow it all the way back to its hive.
- The Ache of Paraguay used excess honey to make sweet beverages – so the first soft drinks were born a long time ago!

SOME SOURCES OF SUGAR IN EARLY HUMAN DIETS

- honey
- insect lerps and galls
- honey ants
- grape sugar
- dates
- maple syrup
- sorghum
- maize
- sugar beets
- sugar cane

In many ways, our present use of refined sugars replaces our previous reliance on honey. In contrast, starches (the other form of carbohydrate energy) played a relatively minor role in human diets until agriculture (growing wheat and corn for example) became our way of life some 10,000 years ago.

Sugars in fruit and honey provided the only carbohydrate energy in human diets for millions of years.

SOURCES OF STARCH

Bread

Breakfast cereals

Rice

Potatoes, potato crisps, chips

Snack foods

Peas

Legumes (dried peas and beans)

Cakes

Biscuits

WHAT *EXACTLY* IS SUGAR?

The term 'sugar' means different things to different people and the terminology can be confusing. In this book, as in everyday language, the word 'sugar' refers to refined cane sugar, unless otherwise indicated. It is by far the main source of refined sugar in British diets.

'Sucrose' is the scientific name for the substance that contributes most of the sweetness in our diet.

The white granular powder extracted from sugar cane that we put in sugar bowls, cakes, biscuits, ice cream and most soft drinks is absolutely identical to the main sugar and source of sweetness in fruit.

Sucrose is chemically classified as a carbohydrate and a simple sugar, specifically a disaccharide composed of glucose and fructose (see diagram).

Glucose   **Fructose**

The chemical structures glucose and fructose.

TYPES OF REFINED SUGAR

White
Brown
Raw
Molasses
Golden syrup
Corn syrup solids
Maltodextrins

The natural sweetness of fruit and honey comes from mixtures of sugar, glucose and fructose. The mild sweetness of milk comes from another disaccharide, lactose, composed of glucose and galactose.

Sucrose

The chemical structure of sucrose (cane sugar).

Because sweetness comes from a mixture of sugars, not just sugar, we use many terms to define the original source:

- naturally-occurring sugars
- refined sugars
- added sugars
- concentrated sugars
- intrinsic sugars and extrinsic sugars

If this confuses you, don't worry – it confuses the experts too!

Sucrose is the scientific name for the substance that contributes most of the sweetness in our diet.

THE RISE OF REFINED SUGAR

Refined sugar is also known as table sugar, cane sugar or beet sugar. Sugar cane was one of the first foods that we began to cultivate deliberately (no prize for guessing why!). Sugar cane was first grown in Papua New Guinea 10,000 years ago, and the practice spread gradually to Egypt (2300 years ago), Arabia (1300 years ago) and Japan (1100 years ago). Sugar beet, the main source of refined sugar in cool climates, was first cultivated in Europe 500 years ago.

Sugar cane and sugar beet have a naturally high content of sugar (about 16 per cent) and have been commercially exploited as concentrated sources of sugar since 1600AD. Unfortunately, slaves were the main source of labour. Prior to this, refined sugar was a rare and expensive commodity and honey was much cheaper.

Sugar consumption increased dramatically in Europe from the second half of the 18th century replacing honey as the major source of sweetness. Our consumption levels peaked around 1900 and have remained, with minor variations, much the same for the past 100 years.

Since 1970, corn syrup solids (glucose syrups made from hydrolysed corn starch) have partially replaced some of the refined sugar in manufactured products, particularly in the USA.

Soft drinks (10–12 per cent sugar) are less concentrated sources of sugar than sugar cane (16 per cent sugar) or sugar beet.

WHAT IS THE CONTRIBUTION OF SUGAR TO OUR TOTAL ENERGY INTAKE?

Sugar is often said to be a concentrated form of energy. But a 200-gram apple containing 10 to 12 per cent natural sugars has the same kilocalorie content as 200 millilitres of soft drink.

Sugar even in its most concentrated form, has only half the kilocalories of the same amount of fat or alcohol.

Other carbohydrates such as starch, glucose and fructose have the same energy content per gram.

Direct estimates of refined sugar intake derived from dietary records show that women consume 40 to 60 grams of sugar a day while men eat a little more (60 to 80 grams) and children a little less (30 to 50 grams).

This means that refined sugars contribute about 10 to 12 per cent of total energy intake in most people's diet. This average level is considered acceptable by health authorities all over the world, including those in Australia, New Zealand, the United States, the United Kingdom and Sweden.

We consume a similar amount of naturally-occurring sugars in fruits and vegetables (ie about 60 grams per day). Together, these two sources of sugars make up half our total carbohydrate intake, the remaining half being starch from breads, cereals and potatoes.

HOW MUCH SUGAR DO WE REALLY EAT?

There is considerable confusion and controversy about how much refined sugar we really eat.

Until 1990, the only figures available for refined sugar consumption were derived from 'apparent' consumption statistics, i.e, (gross production of refined sugar plus imports minus export, wastage and non-food usage). The estimates from calculations like this suggested that the average intake of refined sugar alone was around 125 grams a day.

We now know from actual dietary records that these apparent consumption calculations overestimated true consumption by as much as two to three times. Although there is a tendency to under-report sugar intake during dietary assessment, this can't be responsible for all of the difference between apparent consumption and dietary records. It is likely that sugar wastage and non-food use of sugar is much greater than estimates allow.

The interesting aspect of apparent consumption figures is that Britons have hardly changed their intake of refined sugars over the last 100 years. We eat slightly less these days than in the early 1900s. Back then, home-made lemonade and ginger beer, jams and confectionery, crystallised fruit, cakes and biscuits were the main sources of sugar in the diet.

HOW AND WHY IS SUGAR ADDED TO FOODS

Refined sugar is added to foods for more than just its sweetness. For example, sugar contributes to the bulk and texture of cakes and biscuits and it provides viscosity and 'mouth feel' in beverages such as soft drinks and fruit juices. Sugar is also a powerful preservative and contributes to the long storage life of jams and confectionery.

In frozen products like ice cream, sugar has multiple functions: it acts as an emulsifier, preventing the separation of the water and fat phases; it lowers the freezing point thereby making the product more liquid and 'creamier' at the temperature eaten.

The presence of sugar retards the crystallisation of the lactose in dairy foods and milk chocolate (tiny crystals of lactose feel like sand on the tongue).

In canned fruit, sugar syrups are used to prevent mushiness caused by the osmotic movement of sugar out of the fruit and into the surrounding fluid. Because sugar masks unpleasant flavours, sugar syrups are used as carriers for drugs and medicines, especially for young children who are unable to swallow tablet formulations.

In products like yogurt and coffee it masks the acidity or bitterness and balances the sugar-acid ratio in fruit juices and cordials.

Sugar is also the energy source for fermentation carried

out by microorganisms deliberately added to foods. It is added as food for the yeast in bread-making and beer-making. But it is totally converted to alcohol and other products in the process and therefore not consumed as sugar.

WHAT ABOUT LOW-CALORIE PRODUCTS

The difficulties inherent in producing low-calorie products using intense sweeteners attest to the fact that refined sugar is added to foods for more than just its sweetness.

When manufacturers design a low-calorie, low-sugar product they find that many substances (e.g. preservatives, emulsifiers, antioxidants) need to be added to perform all the roles that sugar did alone.

HOW MUCH HONEY DID OUR ANCESTORS EAT?

It is possible that intakes of honey at various times during history may well have rivalled our current consumption of refined sugar.

In pre-industrial times, honey was the main source of concentrated sweetness in the diets of many peoples. There are no precise figures for their consumption because honey was part of either a hunter/gatherer or subsistence economy. Until recently, historians and food writers have proposed that it was a scarce commodity available only to a wealthy few.

However, a reappraisal of the archaeological evidence from the Stone Age to early Modern times suggests that ordinary people ate much larger quantities of honey than previously thought.

- The Ancient Egyptians made frequent use of honey in their spiced bread, cakes and pastries, and for priming beer and wine.
- In Roman times, half the recipes in a famous cook book call for honey
- In Ancient Greece those who died some distance from home were sometimes preserved in honey in transit.

All of this suggests that there was plenty of honey around. During Medieval times we know that honey was sold in bulk quantities like gallons and even barrels – units unlikely to be used for a scarce commodity. It was present in sufficient abundance to make mead – a common alcoholic drink made from honey.

Even the poorest people could have a beehive because bees often made their homes in a hollow log or a broken pot. Wealthy landowners might own dozens of beautifully constructed beehives and employ a beekeeper.

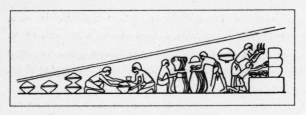

Ancient Egyptians made frequent use of honey

Refined sugar may not have displaced more nutrient-rich items from our present-day diets but only the nutritionally comparable food – honey.

UNDERSTANDING THE SUGAR-FAT SEESAW

In industrialised nations, refined sugar consumption varies from person to person, but there is a consistent relationship between their sugar intake and their fat intake.

As refined sugar intake falls, fat intake rises and vice versa. Those of us who eat the least sugar (expressed as a proportion of our total kilocalorie intake), also eat the most fat, in particular more saturated fat. This is called the 'sugar-fat' seesaw and the relationship has important implications.

Until recently, it was believed that sugar and fat went 'hand-in-hand' and that a diet high in sugar was likely to be high in fat as well. But we now know this is wrong: a high sugar diet is more likely to be low in fat. This evidence has been demonstrated worldwide in adults, teenagers and children; men and women; and in people with diabetes.

VERY FEW PEOPLE ACHIEVE A LOW-FAT DIET WITHOUT INCREASING SUGAR INTAKE

One of the most important implications of the sugar-fat seesaw is that recommendations to reduce both sugar and fat may be counterproductive.

Most people are surprised to learn that the foods which provide most of our sugar intake (e.g. soft drinks, dairy products, breakfast cereals) are very low in fat. Similarly, the foods that provide most of our fat (e.g. meat, butter/margarine, fried foods), are very low in sugar. In fact, only 10 per cent of our kilocalories are in the form of high-fat/high-sugar combinations like ice-cream and chocolate.

You may well be wondering how people in less affluent areas like Africa and China manage without sugar and still manage to eat a low-fat diet.

While it's true that they eat a low-fat, low-sugar diet, their actual diet is far from balanced and optimal – their total energy and micronutrient intake is often lower than it should be, resulting in compromised growth and nutrition. High starch diets are not necessarily a recipe for lifelong health and longevity.

Research shows that reducing your fat intake (especially saturated fat) is certainly more likely to result in desirable changes in body weight, blood lipids, insulin sensitivity and cardiovascular risk factors. But trying to reduce your sugar intake at the same time may not only compromise the effort to reduce fat, but reduce the palatability of the diet and hence the likelihood of sticking to the low-fat diet long term.

High starch diets are not necessarily a recipe for lifelong health and longevity.

DOES SUGAR INCREASE THE RISK OF VITAMIN AND MINERAL DEFICIENCIES?

Refined sugar and other added sugars are regarded by many people as undesirable because they are 'empty calories' – that is, providing energy but without vitamins and minerals.

It's logical to assume that sugar 'dilutes' the vitamin and mineral content of the diet but the real question is whether it happens in practice. If it were true, then we would expect to find that diets containing the least sugar would have the greatest quantities of micronutrients. But many large well-designed scientific studies found this not to be the case. In fact, diets containing moderately large amounts of added sugars were found to be the most nutritious, more so than diets low in sugar or very high in sugar.

This was true in adults, teenagers and young children. In some cases such as vitamin C, vitamin B2 and calcium, it was found that the higher the sugar content of the diet, the higher the intake of the micronutrient.

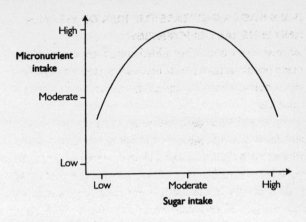

In UK diets, the moderate consumption of sugars is associated with the highest intake of micronutrients.

One of the reasons for this paradox is that sweetened foods can be excellent sources of micronutrients – breakfast cereals and dairy products such as flavoured milk, yogurts and ice cream are good examples. They are more likely to be eaten frequently and in larger quantities when sweetened. Many of us known children who refuse to drink plain milk but tuck into a strawberry milkshake or hot chocolate. A couple of teaspoons of brown sugar on porridge or a dollop of jam on toast encourages us to eat nutritious but otherwise fairly bland foods.

The second reason that moderate sugar intake equates with greater intake of micronutrients is the sugar-fat seesaw that is, low-sugar diets in practice are usually higher in fat. Fats such as cooking oils, butter and margarines are essentially 'empty calories' too. Of course, they do contain some vitamins, particularly the fat-soluble vitamins, but their very high energy content means they tend to dilute rather than enrich the micro-nutrients in the rest of the diet.

THE FATE OF SUGAR IN YOUR BODY

After swallowing, sugar is emptied from the stomach into the small intestine where it undergoes digestion. The enzyme responsible for sugar digestion is called sucrase, located in the lining of the small intestine. The enzyme digests sucrose into glucose and fructose which are then absorbed into the bloodstream. Much of the sugar we add to foods has already been broken down prior to consumption. We actually swallow a mixture of glucose, fructose and sucrose. Soft drinks are a good example.

The glucose molecule derived from sugar digestion is transported rapidly into the bloodstream while fructose is absorbed much more slowly. So slowly, in fact, that a large quantity of fructose (more than 30 grams) by itself will cause diarrhoea. The high fructose content of apple juice has been blamed for 'toddler diarrhoea'.

Once absorbed into the bloodstream, glucose and fructose travel to the liver where some of the glucose and virtually all the fructose is removed. The fructose is burned as an immediate source of energy, while glucose passes into the circulation entering the muscles and other tissues under the influence of the hormone insulin. In the muscle cells, glucose displaces fat as the source of energy and is burned to carbon dioxide and water. Under normal circumstances very little of the glucose is converted to fat.

THE IMPORTANCE OF BLOOD SUGAR

A normal blood sugar (glucose) level is our lifeline. It allows our brains, red cells and other systems to function properly.

If our blood sugar levels drop too low, brain function is compromised and we suffer symptoms such as sweating and nausea.

If blood sugar levels are too high for too long, then eyesight, kidney and heart function are affected. The glucose in our blood is derived from our diet as well as synthesis in the liver.

BLOOD SUGAR OR BLOOD GLUCOSE?

Blood sugar and blood glucose mean exactly the same thing. In this book we use the term blood sugar because it is the one most familiar to the public.

Consuming sugar (and any other carbohydrate including starch) produces hormonal responses which help the body take up the new source of energy and also limit the rise in blood sugar levels.

Insulin plays an important role in bringing blood sugar levels back to normal after the meal by 'opening the gates' and transporting glucose from the blood into the cells. Since there is plenty of glucose around, insulin also switches off the synthesis of new glucose molecules in the liver and also the breakdown of fat as a source of energy.

During the 3–4 hours after a meal, the amount of carbohydrate consumed (whether as starch or sugar) far exceeds the amount of carbohydrate that can be oxidised in the cells. As a result, much of the dietary carbohydrate-derived glucose is stored as glycogen in the liver and skeletal muscles and is subsequently released and oxidised within the next 12 hours.

Thus the fate of sugar in your body is the same as all other dietary carbohydrates:

- oxidation (burning) in the tissues as a source of energy
- storage as glycogen in liver and muscle cells
- recycling in the liver for the synthesis of new glucose molecules (this is quite an active pathway)
- conversion and storage as fat mainly in the liver (under unusual circumstances only)

The body's glycogen reserves are small (usually 250 to 500 grams in a 50- to 70-kilogram adult, higher in trained athletes). The capacity to store more can be developed by exercise, training and diet.

A normal diet provides about 200 to 300 grams of carbohydrate a day. Thus within any 24-hour period, there is total oxidation of absorbed dietary carbohydrate, including sugar. Other metabolic pathways for disposal of dietary carbohydrate, such as conversion into fat or non-essential amino acids, are relatively unimportant in comparison.

BLOOD SUGAR RESPONSES AFTER A MEAL

After a meal containing sugar or starch, the plasma glucose rises reaching a peak within 15 to 30 minutes and returns to baseline within 2 hours. In people with diabetes, this peak occurs later – between 45 and 60 minutes after the meal because there is a relative deficiency of insulin. In the past, it was assumed that refined sugar caused a more rapid rise in blood glucose levels than starchy foods or naturally occurring sources of sugars like fruit. This assumption has been shown to be incorrect.

Most starchy foods, including potatoes, bread and many breakfast cereals are digested and absorbed rapidly and the blood sugar response is almost as high as that seen with an equivalent load of pure glucose. Foods containing refined sugar, such as soft drinks and ice cream have been shown to give moderate rises in blood sugar, on average less than that of bread.

Additionally, the blood sugar response to foods containing refined sugars is similar to that of foods containing natural-occurring sugars.

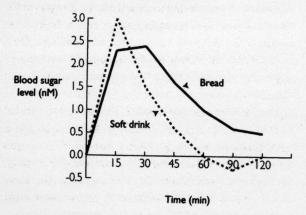

Comparison of blood sugar responses after 50 grams of carbohydrate in the form of sucrose or bread. Although soft drink raises blood sugar to a higher level momentarily (at 15 minutes), it declines quickly. In contrast, bread raises blood sugar levels for longer. From 30 minutes onwards blood sugar levels are higher after consuming bread.

THE GLYCAEMIC INDEX OF FOODS (THE G.I. FACTOR)

The glycaemic index or G.I. factor is used to classify foods according to their ability to raise the level of sugars in the blood. Foods are tested in equivalent carbohydrate portions according to standardised methodology. On a scale where glucose equals 100, the G.I. factor of refined sugar (equals 65) is similar to that of white bread (equals 70).

In a study of over 300 people with diabetes, the overall G.I. of the diet correlated inversely with the percentage of carbohydrate consumed as sugars. The higher the sugars from all sources (both refined and naturally-occurring), the *lower* the overall diet G.I. This result shocks many people, but it results directly from the fact that most common starchy foods, even wholemeal versions, have a high G.I. factor.

Why is this so? Well, if you look back to page 9 you can see that half of the sugar molecule is fructose and half is glucose. Fructose has little effect on blood sugar levels. Starch, on the other hand, is made up of strings of glucose molecules. So gram for gram, sugar contains only half the glucose molecules of starch.

When we consume 50 grams of starch as potatoes, we eat the equivalent of 50 grams of glucose (the starch is rapidly digested to glucose in the small intestine). When we eat 50 grams of sucrose, we eat the equivalent of only 25 grams of glucose, irrespective of the rate of digestion. Hence it's no surprise really that the effect on blood sugar of 25 grams of glucose will be much lower than that of 50 grams of starch or glucose equivalents.

Is this reciprocal relationship between the amount of sugar eaten and the overall G.I. of the diet such a big deal? Well, yes! The researchers also found that glycosylated haemoglobin levels in the blood (the best measure of diabetes control) were found to be correlated directly with the G.I. of the diet. Those with the lowest G.I. (ie those with higher sugar intake) had the best diabetes control.

This goes against much of what is currently preached about sugar and diabetes by many health professionals. Our message of allowing yourself a moderate amount of sugar in your diet (ie the average level eaten by the population) is backed up by dozens of studies showing that sugar does not compromise diabetes control.

The tables on the next 4 pages show the G.I. factor of a range of common foods.

GLYCAEMIC INDEX TABLES FOR SUGAR AND ENERGY

Foods containing refined sugar	G.I.
BAKERY GOODS	
Angel food cake	67
Apple muffin	44
Blueberry muffin	59
Banana cake	47
SWEET BISCUITS	
Digestive plain	59
Oatmeal	55
Milk Arrowroot	69
Morning coffee	79
Rich Tea Cake	55
Shredded Wheat	62
Shortbread	64
Vanilla Wafer	77
BREAKFAST CEREALS	
All-Bran™	42
Cheerios™	74
Cocopops™	77
Cornflakes	84
Muesli, toasted	43
Muesli, non-toasted	56
Rice Bubbles	83
DAIRY FOODS	
Ice Cream – full fat	61
Ice Cream – low fat	50
Milk – chocolate low fat	32
Custard	43
Yoghurt, low fat, fruit	33
CONFECTIONERY	
Jelly Beans	80
Mars Bar™	68
Milk Chocolate	49
SPORTS DRINKS	
Gatorade	78
Sportsplus	74
Isostar	73

SOFT DRINKS

Fanta	68
Coca Cola	63
Orange cordial	66

SPREADS

Nutella™	33
Jams	48–51

Foods with naturally-occurring sugars   G.I.

Apple	38
Apple juice	40
Apricots – fresh	57
Apricots – dried	31
Banana	55
Cherries	22
Dates, dried	103
Grapefruit	25
Grapefruit juice – unsweetened	48
Grapes, green	46
Kiwi fruit	52
Mango	55
Orange	44
Orange juice	46
Paw paw	58
Peach	42
Pear	30
Pineapple	66
Pineapple juice – unsweetened	44
Plums	39
Raisins	64
Sultanas	56
Watermelon	72

Starchy foods (with little or no sugar)   G.I.

BREADS

Dark rye, Schinkebröt	86
French baguette	95
Fruit loaf	47
Hamburger bun	61
Light rye	68
Pitta bread	57
Pumpernickel	41
Rye bread	65

Sourdough, rye	57
White	70
Wholemeal	69

CEREAL GRAINS

Barley, pearled	25
Buckwheat	54
Bulgur, cooked	48
Couscous, cooked	65

Maize

Cornmeal, whole grain	68
Sweet corn, canned	55
Taco shells	68
Millet	71

Rice

Basmati, white	58
Basmati	58
Instant	87
Brown	76
Tapioca, boiled with milk	81

CRACKERS

Wheat crackers	67
Premium soda crackers	74
Puffed crispbread, 20g	81
Rice cakes	82
Ryvita™	69
Water cracker	78

PASTA

Capellini	45
Fettucini	32
Gnocchi	68
Noodles, 2-minute	46
Linguine thick	46
Linguine	55
Macaroni	45
Macaroni and Cheese	64
Ravioli, meat filled	39
Rice pasta, brown	92
Spaghetti – white	41
Spaghetti – wholemeal	37
Spirali durum	43
Star Pastina	38
Tortellini (cheese)	50
Vermicelli	35

POTATOES

Instant potato	83
New	78
New, canned	65
Desirée, boiled	101
French fries	75

LEGUMES AND BEANS

Soya Beans, canned	14
Lima Beans baby, frozen	32
Lentils – green and brown, boiled	30
Lentils – red, boiled	26
Black Beans, boiled	30
Black Gram, soaked and boiled	43
Butter Beans, boiled	31
Chickpeas, canned/drained	42
Chickpeas, boiled	33
Haricot (Navy Beans), boiled	38
Split Peas – yellow, boiled	32

SNACKS

Potato crisps	57
Pretzels	83

SO WHAT DO THE EXPERTS SAY ABOUT SUGAR AND HEALTH?

Sugar's overall effect on health has been studied by experts in many countries. The FAO/WHO group concluded that:

■ Moderate intake of sugar-rich foods can provide for a palatable and nutritious diet.

The American panel concluded that:

■ At the levels normally consumed sugar has no effect on disease risk, apart from dental decay.

The British committee came to similar conclusions but were more cautious in their recommendations.

The Australian Panel agreed with the consensus of opinion all around the world that:

■ Refined sugar should contribute no more than 12 per cent of energy to the diet.

What does this mean for you?

Well, this means about 60 grams (3 tablespoons) of sugar per day from sources including soft drinks, breakfast cereals and bakery products. At present, the average level of consumption in Western countries meets this target.

Of course, there are people that eat more than this – indeed, some eat as much as 120 grams a day but they are often the people who can afford to, and even need a non-bulky source of carbohydrate energy – very active teenage males, heavy labourers and endurance athletes.

The difficulty is that the public and some health authorities, however, remain concerned about health effect of sugars especially in relation to diabetes and dental disease.

Don't go overboard!

Our intention in this little book is not to suggest you should indulge in an excessive amount of sugar simply because sugar restriction is unnecessary. Far from it! But we do want to take the pressure off. We want you to feel that your normal instincts will guide you to eat a moderate quantity of sugar – the amount that is eaten by the average consumer – about 60 grams of refined sugar per day.

To give you a guide to what this means in practice we have provided the following menu. We also list the refined sugar content of a range of common foods.

Guidelines for usual intake of refined sugars

Women 40–60 g/day
Men 60–80 g/day
Children 30–50 g/day

A one-day menu containing a moderate quantity of sugar

Breakfast
2 Weetabix™ with low fat milk
and 2 teaspoons sugar
2 slices wholegrain toast with margarine
and honey (20 g)
Coffee with low fat milk and
1 teaspoon of sugar

Snack
2 sweet biscuits
White tea

Lunch
Ham and salad sandwich on grain bread
An apple
250 ml orange juice

Snack
A pear
Glass of water

Dinner
Steak with potato, peas, carrots and corn
2 scoops low fat ice-cream
with 1 tablespoon of chocolate topping
Coffee with low fat milk
and 1 teaspoon sugar

Snack
3 squares of chocolate
Coffee with low fat milk
and 1 teaspoon sugar

This menu contains 60 grams of added sugar.

The menu on pages 39–40 provides 1900 kcal and meets the recommended proportions of nutrients, with 24 per cent energy coming from fat (Recommendation: <30 per cent) and 57 per cent of energy coming from carbohydrate (Recommendation: >50 per cent).

The total carbohydrate content is 285g made up of 123 g starch + 155 g sugars (60 g added, 95 g naturally occurring).

A moderate quantity of sugar in a 10-year-old child's diet

Breakfast
½ cup of Coco-Pops™ with reduced fat milk
½ banana
100 ml of fruit juice

Snack
1 small apple
1 cup of home-made popcorn
A cup of reduced fat milk

Lunch
½ cup of egg noodles with grated cheese
1 mini corn cob
A cup of water

Snack
4 dried apricot halves
2 chocolate chip biscuits
A glass of cordial

Dinner
½ cup spaghetti with meat sauce
Carrot and celery sticks
½ cup custard and a canned pear half
Water to drink

This child's menu provides 50 grams of refined sugars. It provides 1500 kcal energy with 25 per cent of energy from fat and 58 per cent of energy from carbohydrate.

A low G.I. menu for someone with diabetes containing a moderate quantity of sugar

Breakfast
1 cup of rolled oats with low fat milk
and a dessertspoon of brown sugar
A fresh orange
Tea or coffee with low fat milk

Snack
2 Ginger Biscuits
Tea or coffee with low fat milk

Lunch
A mixed grain sandwich filled with
avocado, carrot, beetroot, tomato and lettuce
200 g low-fat fruit yoghurt
Glass of water

Dinner
Pan-fried fish with spinach, tomato and onion
served over a cup of rice
Tea or coffee with low fat milk

Snack
2 scoops low fat ice cream
with canned pears

This menu contains 40 g of added sugar. The total energy content is 1525 kcal. 22 per cent of energy is from fat, 55 per cent from carbohydrate. The fat content is 38 g. The total carbohydrate content is 220 grams, with 112 grams from starch and 108 grams from sugars (added plus naturally occurring).

REFINED SUGAR CONTENT OF VARIOUS FOODS (GRAMS)

1 rounded teaspoon of sugar	6
1 tablespoon of jam	8
1 tablespoon of honey	20
1 boiled lolly	5
5 squares chocolate	20
1 chocolate bar (average)	35
375 ml can of soft drink (average)	45
1 cup of sweetened fruit juice	5
30 ml undiluted cordial	18
1 muesli bar (average)	8
1 shortbread biscuit	3
1 cream filled biscuit	5
1 piece of chocolate cake	11
1 cinnamon and sugar doughnut	7
1 piece of plain cake	7

SOURCES OF REFINED SUGARS

Soft drinks, cordials and fruit juice drinks
Sweetened dairy products (ice cream, yogurt, flavoured milk, custard)
Milk flavourings (Nesquik™)
Sweetened breakfast cereals
Flavoured toppings
Jams, honey, golden syrup, Nutella™
Cakes, biscuits and bakery products
Confectionery and chocolate
Ice blocks and frozen confections
Table sugars – white, raw, brown, castor, cube

Sources of naturally-occurring sugars

Fruit of any sort
Honey
Dried fruit (dates, sultanas, raisins)
Breast milk (lactose)
Cow's milk (lactose)
Vegetables (some are higher than others, e.g. carrots, peppers, tomatoes, sweet corn, sugarbeet)

IS THERE SUCH A THING AS SUGAR-CRAVING?

The notion that we can become addicted to sugar and crave it constantly is based on the false assumption that sugar causes wild fluctuations in blood sugar – that it sends blood sugars soaring, floods the system with sugar and creates rebound or reactive 'hypoglycaemia' (low blood sugar levels). The low blood sugars are claimed to be responsible for the 'craving'.

This simply isn't true. Many studies show that most sugary foods cause very moderate rises in blood sugar. Bread and potatoes produce higher blood sugar levels than sugar and no-one ever hears about potato addiction!

If we crave sugar, it's because we humans have an instinctive liking for it – part of the hard wiring in the brain that tells us that a food that is sweet is a safe form of energy. If we deny this instinct by deliberately restricting sweet food, it's not surprising that it creates a 'no-win' situation.

Studies of people who claimed to crave sugar, actually found that the preferred foods were sweet-fat combinations such as cakes and biscuits, which contain more energy as fat than they do as sugar.

Women appear to like these sweet-fat combinations more than men whose preference is for meat and starch-fat combinations like baked potatoes. This female preference may be related to a woman's greater requirement for carbohydrate during pregnancy and lactation. The foetus uses only glucose as a source of fuel (fat can't cross the placenta) and is entirely dependent on the mother for this glucose. During lactation, women secrete up to 70 grams of carbohydrate a day in the form of the sugar in milk.

So, if you think you have a sugar craving, you don't have to beat it or bust it. Enjoy!

If you have a sugar craving
you don't have to beat it
or bust it. Enjoy!

DOES SUGAR PROMOTE CANDIDA AND THRUSH (YEAST) INFECTIONS?

Many natural health therapists claim that high-sugar diets promote the growth of yeast infections of the vagina, mouth and skin. While infections caused by Candida albicans are very common, there is absolutely no evidence that a diet high in sugars causes the infection or influences it in any way.

The Candida organism is in our bodies all the time. The infection comes from its uncontrolled growth often caused by the use of antibiotics which inhibit the bacteria that normally control yeast numbers. Symptoms of excessive growth are itching and burning sensations.

One of the reasons sugar is often heard in connection with Candida is that people with diabetes are particularly prone to infection with this organism. When blood sugars are abnormally high, as in uncontrolled diabetes, the sugars spill over into the urine and create a good medium for the growth of the organism. But because starches increase blood sugars to the same or greater extent than sugary foods, potatoes and bread would be incriminated in Candida infections too!

WHAT ABOUT SUGAR AND DIABETES?

Diabetes associations worldwide have now recognised that there is no need to strictly avoid refined sugar. This change of heart resulted from the unarguable scientific evidence that blood sugar responses after eating sugary foods were no higher than that of starchy staples such as bread.

In longer term studies in people with diabetes, those who were required to eat 50 grams a day of refined sugar in tea and coffee had no higher average blood sugars than those assigned to artificial sweeteners. Even extremely large amounts of sugar (300 grams a day) did not compromise blood sugar control – but this amount is definitely not recommended! It just proves a point.

There is no evidence to suggest that refined sugar causes worsening of glucose tolerance, insulin sensitivity or diabetes risk in humans. There are studies in rats that support this idea but the amounts of sugar fed to the rats (equivalent to 100 or more cans of soft drink a day) are so much higher than a human would ever eat or want to eat, that the findings are really irrelevant. When rats are fed sugar at the upper levels of human consumption, no adverse effects have been noted.

The important point is that avoiding sugar has consequences of its own that can be far more serious than any potential effects of eating refined sugar. In other words, restricting sugar may actually be counterproductive in people with diabetes. This is because of the sugar-fat seesaw and the fact that starchy foods are often high G.I.

Past studies in people with diabetes have clearly shown they eat less sugar but more saturated fat than the general population. The consequence, of course, is that they die of heart disease caused by hardening of the arteries. Some of our readers might be saying that we should all try harder to restrict both sugar and fat, but this means starchy foods must increase to fill the gap.

The trouble is that there are good and bad starchy foods. If starchy foods with a high G.I. factor such as bread and potatoes, fill the hole left by sugar, then it may do more harm than good. Unlike sugar, high G.I. starchy foods have been associated with increasing the risk of diabetes and heart disease in the general population.

Two large studies from Harvard School of Public Health involving 65,000 female nurses and 50,000 male health professionals, showed that diets with a high G.I.

factor and low dietary fibre content were associated with a doubling of the risk of type 2 diabetes. In the Nurses' Study, there was a doubling of the risk of heart attack in those consuming a high G.I. diet. The harmful consequences for people with diabetes are likely to be greater still.

Unlike sugar, high G.I. starchy foods have been associated with increasing the risk of diabetes and heart disease in <u>the general population</u>.

WHAT ABOUT SUGAR AND BLOOD CHOLESTEROL?

Most readers will be aware that high blood cholesterol levels increase our risk of a heart attack. The dietary component most clearly associated with increasing cholesterol levels is saturated fat. Reducing saturated fat is the most effective way to reduce the risk of heart attack.

Sugar, on the other hand, has never been found to increase cholesterol levels. When we reduce saturated fat, carbohydrate energy increases to replace the missing kilocalories. In some studies, this increase in carbohydrate intake – either from starches or sugars – has been found to cause a rise in blood triglyceride levels and a fall in the 'good' form of cholesterol, HDL. Together these two trends are not desirable because they can act independently of cholesterol levels to increase our risk of heart disease.

This is especially true in people with diabetes, who more often than not, have a high risk of heart disease despite normal blood cholesterol levels. As a result, some experts suggest that the best course of action is to avoid both saturated fat and large amounts of carbohydrate and eat monounsaturated fat instead.

This is the reasoning behind the promotion of diets high in olive oil. Indeed, people in Mediterranean countries who do eat more unsaturated fat and less carbohydrate than other industrialised countries have a low risk of heart disease. But their diet and lifestyle differ in many other ways that may act in unison to reduce heart disease risk.

They eat more fruit and vegetables, more pasta and legumes, more salads and vinaigrette dressings. All of these foods have a low G.I. factor, so that blood sugars are as low as possible and the tendency of carbohydrate to increase blood triglycerides and reduce HDL is reduced. Olive oil alone is not responsible for the reduced risk of heart disease in Mediterranean countries.

Some nutrition experts are concerned that diets high in sugar might increase blood triglycerides more so than with other carbohydrates. The basis of this worry is that studies incorporating very large amounts of sugars (providing one-third or more of total kilocalories) have found higher blood triglycerides and lower HDL than when starch was eaten.

Furthermore, some people appear to be more sensitive to the effects of dietary sugars on blood fats than are others. We do not yet know the reason for this variation among individuals but it is clear that people with diabetes are not among the sensitive ones.

This is one area where we need more research before we can be absolutely clear about the role of sugar. In the meantime, however, you can be reassured that diets that contain more typical amounts of sugar (around 50 to 60 grams a day or 12 per cent energy), have no special effect on blood fats.

When we reduce saturated fat, carbohydrate energy increases to replace the missing kilocalories.

DOES SUGAR MAKE YOU FAT?

There is a widespread belief that sugar is particularly associated with weight gain and obesity. This view stems largely from early studies in rats and mice which showed water sweetened with sugar led to rapid weight gain – not really surprising because water laced with any form of energy whether it be amino acids, starch or fat would do the same thing. Milk causes rapid weight gain too! But the deed was done and sugar's reputation for causing exceptional weight gain was accepted by the public and scientific community at large.

It's become clear that rats and humans are very different in respect to fat-making enzymes. Rodents are very efficient in converting carbohydrates like sugar or starch into fat in the body, while humans have only limited quantities of the necessary enzymes and do it only under unusual circumstances.

Human fat stores have been created by channelling excess fat energy to fat storage, not by converting excess carbohydrate into fat. We know this because our fat stores have the very same fatty acid composition as our diet. If our diet is high in monounsaturated fat, then our fat stores will reflect this.

If we eat an excessive amount of carbohydrate energy, some of it will be stored as glycogen in our liver and muscles and all of it will eventually be burnt (oxidised) as a fuel source.

If we overeat a very high carbohydrate diet (which is rather hard to do because it's often bulky and very satiating), then it is the small amount of fat in the diet that will be channelled to fat storage.

Even an exceedingly large meal of pure glucose (500 grams, the equivalent of 5 litres of soft drink in one hit) does not induce a net gain in fat. If overfeeding of glucose extends for several days, glycogen stores do become full (at about 1000 grams) and only at this point does sugar convert to fat. But this artificial situation is unlikely to occur outside the laboratory.

In everyday life, a high intake of sugars induces an increase in satiety, and subsequently food intake is decreased.

One of the most robust findings in recent nutrition science is that sugars result in much greater feelings of fullness compared to high-fat meals containing the same number of kilocalories.

In one study, students ate as much as they liked from a

palatable smorgasbord of either high-sugar foods or high-fat foods on two separate occasions. They were 'blind' to the nutrient content of the foods and the true purpose of the study. The investigators found that the students consumed far fewer kilocalories overall when they ate from the smorgasbord of high sugar foods.

In another study, students were given either a high-sugar or a high-fat snack and 1 hour later allowed to eat from an array of palatable foods. They ate significantly less when the earlier snack was high in sugars.

Scientists now say that fat is very easy to 'passively over-consume'. Of course a high-fat meal can make you feel full, even biliously full. But the point is that you will have eaten an excessively large number of kilocalories before you register this. We all know that it's all too easy to keep munching on those more-ish high fat foods like chips and peanuts.

But we tend not to do the same thing with high sugar foods – eating jelly beans and other sugar confectionery is much more self-limiting – many of us feel a little nauseous if we indulge to excess.

The final test of the theory that 'sugar makes you fat' is to look at the association between sugar intake and body weight in the general population. It's important that we exclude the dieters from such studies because they will tend to muddle the interpretation of the findings, having altered their diet in an effort to lose weight.

A well-designed study involving over 10,000 Scottish adults showed that diets low in sugars were associated with higher body mass index (a measure of overweight). In contrast, the diets high in sugars were associated with lower body weight. In fact, there was a consistent stepwise relationship between the two factors – the higher the sugar intake as a percentage of energy or in grams per day, the lower the body mass index. This applied to both refined sugar and total sugars from all sources. This did not apply to starch – there was no difference in starch intake in lean and overweight people.

In a recent Australian study of identical twins, there was little to associate any dietary factor with the degree of overweight. But, when the twins differed in weight by more than 4 kilograms, the lighter twin tended to have a diet higher in sugar than the heavier twin.

Many other studies can be cited which show this inverse association between sugars and weight status. All of them are open to the criticism that conscious or unconscious 'under-reporting' of sugar by the heaviest people is responsible for the trend. However, the same can be said of fat under-reporting and yet fat shows a direct relationship to body weight in the same studies.

There is ample reason to incriminate high-fat diets with overweight (passive overconsumption being one!), but no good scientific evidence to point the finger at sugar.

'There is no evidence of a direct involvement of sucrose, other sugars and starch in the etiology of lifestyle-related diseases.'

—United Nations FAO/WHO
Expert Consultation on Carbohydrates, 1998

EFFECT OF SUGAR ON BEHAVIOUR

The belief that sugar causes ADD (attention deficit disorder, previously known as hyperactivity) is based on two theories:

- a possible allergic response
- a low blood sugar 'rebound' after sugar consumption

However, results from many published studies representing hundreds of subjects do not provide any support whatsoever for the idea that refined sugar causes or exacerbates ADD or affects cognitive performance in children. Even those children originally considered to be adversely affected by sugar showed no effects when the sugar was given in a situation where neither the investigator or child or parent knew the content of the capsules or food.

It is possible that a very tiny number of children may have idiosyncratic reactions and may respond adversely to sugar. However, any carbohydrate, including bread and potatoes, will also be incriminated if the effect is mediated via fluctuations in blood sugar.

There is some evidence that sugar might actually have a calming effect, if it has any effect at all.

Glucose or sugar is known to influence the distress associated with painful procedures in human infants. In one study there was a reduction in crying and heart rate in infants subjected to heel prick when they were given a 50 per cent sugar solution immediately prior to the procedure as compared with control children who were given water.

There is some evidence that sugar may have a calming effect, if it has any effect at all.

WHAT IS THE EFFECT OF SUGAR ON MEMORY?

There is growing evidence that glucose consumption enhances learning and memory in both rats and humans. The effect is best demonstrated in elderly people and those with Alzheimer's, but is also seen in young adults, if the test is sufficiently difficult.

In one study, elderly people were given a battery of neuropsychological tests measuring memory, overall intelligence, attention and motor functions after consuming a lemon-flavoured drink sweetened with either 50 grams of glucose or saccharin. Glucose enhanced performance on the logical and verbal memory part of the tests but there was no effect on attention.

In university students, glucose increased memory for narrative prose with 40 per cent greater recall.

IS SUGAR RELATED IN ANY WAY TO CANCER?

In the United Kingdom, a recent major report of an expert group on nutritional aspects of the development of cancer, hardly mentions sugar at all. In the 15 pages of conclusions and recommendations, two sentences include the word sugars as one of a group of 'other nutrients' along with starch, folates, selenium, calcium, iron and zinc which might have to be involved in the causation or prevention of some cancers. The working party comments that there is not enough evidence to reach conclusions – either positive or negative for any of these substances.

The Committee recommended a balanced diet rich in cereals, fruit and vegetables. Sugar, when consumed within these dietary guidelines is not implicated in cancer causation.

SUGAR AND DENTAL DECAY

Much of what we know about the relationship of sugars to dental decay was gathered before the 'fluoride era'. Sugar's bad reputation was consolidated at that time when research showed a strong relationship between the number of decayed and missing teeth and the amount of sugar eaten.

In the post-fluoride era, it is clear that the best way to promote healthy teeth is to drink fluoridated water, brush your teeth twice a day and use a fluoridated toothpaste. Total sugar consumption has less to do with it than we once thought. Nowadays dentists recognise that all fermentable carbohydrates, i.e. both sugars and starches, can promote dental decay. More importantly, it is not the total amount eaten, but the frequency of eating and consistency of the food that determine its cariogenic potential. Fortunately, fluoride has dramatically reduced the risk of decay even among those with inappropriate eating patterns.

Australian monitoring surveys of child dental health have documented substantial and continuing reductions in dental decay since the 1970s. Capital cities in Australia began to fluoridate their water supplies in 1964. Brisbane is the only non-fluoridated capital city. Dental decay experience in 12-year-old children declined from approximated 8 teeth per child in 1965 to 1 tooth per child in 1995. The report says that total sugar consumption has not played a substantial role in the reduction in decay experience. On the other hand, tooth brushing with fluoride and lifetime exposure to fluoridated water show strong relationships to the number of decayed and missing teeth.

—Australian Institute of Health and Welfare 'Australia's Health 1998'

In Australia, children exposed to fluoride all their lives have little or no dental decay despite high sugar intake. In Britain there has been a similar effect. Some people think fluoride is a poison that ought not be used at all, but there is evidence that humans evolved in parts of the world where water was naturally fluoridated and that we are therefore dependent on small amounts for a healthy set of teeth.

Of course, excessive fluoride is undesirable and children who eat the toothpaste can show white patches on their teeth as a result. Although this might look unsightly, it does no harm. New children's toothpastes with lower levels of fluoride help to prevent this. Your dentist will give advice based on local levels of fluoride in water.

All fermentable carbohydrates, including sugars and starches, are capable of causing holes in the teeth. Naturally-occurring sugars in breast milk, fruit and honey are no different from those in confectionery. Whole grain cereals and flours are just as culpable. The starches in bread, breakfast cereals and potatoes, when caught between the teeth, are risk factors in the initiation of dental decay. Thus, it makes no sense to single out sugar for reduction, while simultaneously recommending higher starch intake.

Indeed, the first archaeological evidence of dental decay appeared 10,000 years ago when humans first adopted farming and starch became a common component of the diet (and long before refined sugar came along). Even in those days some people lost all their teeth to dental decay.

Mechanisms of dental decay

Every meal time and every time we eat or drink, we subject our teeth to an unavoidable 'acid wash'. This is because the bacteria in plaque ferment the residual carbohydrate that remains on teeth to acid.

Acid formation begins within minutes of eating and gradually dissolves the enamel of the surface of the teeth. Teeth strengthened by fluoride have the best defence against this acid. Foods like cornflakes can produce just as much acid as sugary foods. Over the next half hour, the acids are gradually neutralised by saliva and the tooth surface returns to normal.

Dental experts have shown that our teeth can put up with around six of these 'acid washes' a day and still stay in good shape. If you eat all your fermentable carbohydrates at breakfast, morning tea, lunch, afternoon tea, dinner and supper, then your teeth should theoretically stay decay-free.

However, sticky foods like lollies that remain on the

teeth or stuck between teeth for long periods promote tooth decay because the acids are continually being formed by bacterial fermentation. Lollies are not the only culprit however – dried fruit can stick between teeth too! Similarly, if we sip sweet drinks for hours (whether soft drink or juice), we prolong the acid bath and increase the risk of holes.

Some babies develop severe tooth decay by being continuously breast-fed or bottle-fed through-out the night. If we eat very frequently, whether it be non-sugary foods like potato chips or naturally-occurring sugary foods like fruit, we promote acid formation and dental decay. In one study, dental decay was found to be significantly greater in citrus and other fruit-pickers compared to the neighbouring workers on vegetable farms.

Confectionery promotes dental decay because it's more likely to be confectionery than any other food product that's eaten between meals. Furthermore, many types of confectionery take a long time to dissolve in the mouth (e.g. barley sugar), are sticky (chews, liquorice) or are sucked for long periods (lollipops). There is no doubt that frequent consumption of these types of food will promote tooth decay even in fluoridated areas. The actual amount of sugar eaten may be quite small, but the effect is enormous.

If we decide to replace these between meal snacks with more 'natural' products such as dried fruit, or with starchy foods such as bread and crackers, we may be no better off. It all comes down to frequency of consumption between meals.

The unlucky minority in Australia that still suffer severe dental decay tend to be from socio-economic groups where fluoride exposure (both before and after birth) has been lower and a toothbrush is rarely used. Raising socio-economic status will have long-term benefits on both teeth and general health, irrespective of sugar intake.

Strategies to reduce dental decay are far more likely to be successful if the emphasis is placed on fluoridated toothpastes and good dental hygiene, rather than reduction in consumption of sugars.

Regular tooth brushing plays a more important role in the prevention of tooth decay in the post-fluoride era.

A word about low-calorie soft drinks

Low-calorie soft drinks in place of regular varieties are one of the most frequent ways that people endeavour to reduce their sugar intake. If the intention here is to reduce dental decay, then this is not the way to do it. Low-calorie soft drinks are highly acidic, just like regular soft drinks and most fruits. The acidic nature of the solution helps to dissolve the enamel on the tooth surface, even in the absence of bacteria and plaque. We've all heard the story of one famous brand of soft drink that completely dissolved a tooth overnight. Well the same will happen with the regular or diet version of any soft drink.

The present fashion to carry and drink water (both free and expensive versions) instead of juice or soft drink is a good trend. Many people, much of the time, walk around in a state of semi-dehydration that affects both mental and physical performance!

GOOD INTENTIONS

One of the main messages of this little book is that well-intentioned efforts to reduce sugar intake may do more harm than good. Conscious and unconscious reduction in sugar intake is usually accompanied by increases in the intake of foods with a high G.I. factor such as bread and rice, or foods with high levels of saturated fat such as cheese, crackers and potato crisps. Such foods may do more long-term harm to health than sugar ever will.

While many nutritionists feel that people ought to be able to reduce both sugar and fat to low levels, only a small minority of the population actually does so in practice. Furthermore, this recommendation is based on the assumed superiority of starches to sugars – that high intake of starchy foods like cereals, bread and potatoes always coincides with the best of health. Unfortunately, this is not necessarily so – populations all over the world that have high intakes of starch are among those with the highest rates of protein-energy malnutrition and growth stunting. Furthermore, starchy foods with a high G.I., increase insulin demand and therefore promote the diseases of affluence – diabetes, heart disease and obesity. Sugary foods have a lower G.I. than most starchy foods.

Emphasis on reducing sugar intake also fuels the demand for intense sweeteners to use as sugar substitutes. In China, the relatively new soft drink industry is based almost entirely on saccharin-sweetened drinks because sugar is more expensive in China and seen as something that ought best to be avoided. While there is no evidence that intense sweeteners cause harm, there is actually little support for using them at all. In theory, we avoid kilocalories by choosing them, but inevitably we 'catch up' or compensate later in one way or another. Britain is still an overweight nation despite the number of low-calorie products that are on the market.

Millions of pounds are spent on the research and development, safety testing and product development of foods incorporating intense sweeteners. In our opinion, this money would be better channelled to research on the real causes of obesity and diabetes and their treatment.

There may be a place for tooth-friendly confectionery based on sugar substitutes that can be eaten frequently without causing harm. Intense sweeteners are probably here to stay simply because nutrition and other health authorities continue to push the message that sugar is to be avoided if at all possible.

Sugar can be used to maximise your well-being and enjoyment of life.

Our take-home message is that average levels of sugar consumption (around 50–60 grams a day in a typical diet) should be encouraged. It is associated with:

- the highest intake of micronutrients
- lower intakes of saturated fat
- a diet with a lower G.I.
- a lower body weight

You don't need to beat it or bust it,
and you can cut the guilt trip.
The desire for sweetness in foods is a human one.

Use sugar to increase your intake of those very nutritious but rather bland foods – low-fat milk, yogurt, porridge and other wholegrain breakfast cereals. Don't hesitate to put a dollop of jam on your bread, a tablespoon of honey on your wheat biscuits, sprinkle sugar on unripe, sour or acidic fruit, and sweeten carrots and peas with a little sugar.

Don't fret about the sugar in baked beans or canned fruit – these foods are good for you and if you are more likely to eat them because you like them sweetened, go ahead and enjoy.

In the supermarket, pass up the 'no added sugar' products. If soft drink is something that gives you a lot of pleasure, drink it in moderation but don't forget your five servings of fruits and vegetables. If ice cream is your weak spot, choose low-fat, not low sugar versions. If you want to 'pig out' now and again – much better to do it on jelly beans and sugar confectionery than chocolate and potato chips.

EXERCISE AS PART OF YOUR LIFESTYLE

It is important to be as active as possible. The more active you are the more you can afford to indulge your natural desire for sweetness, so make exercise a normal part of your life – walk to the station, use the stairs, give the dog a treat, shoot a few balls with the kids. You don't need to join expensive gyms or do aerobics if that's not your cup of tea. There's a lot of truth in that advertisement.

Exercise – take it regularly, not seriously.

WHERE TO GO FOR FURTHER HELP

British Dietetic Association
5th Floor, Elizabeth House
22 Suffolk Street
Queensway
Birmingham, B1 1LS
Telephone: 0121 616 4900

REFERENCES

1. Asp N-G. Nutritional classification and analysis of carbohydrates. American Journal of Clinical Nutrition 1994;59(suppl):679S–681S.
2. Wursch P. Starch in human nutrition. World Review of Nutrition and Dietetics 1989;60:199–256.
3. Baghurst KI, Baghurst PA, Record SJ. Demographic and nutritional profiles of people consuming varying levels of added sugars. Nutrition Research 1992;12:1455–1465.
4. Gibson SA. Consumption and sources of sugars in the diets of British schoolchildren: are high sugar diets nutritionally inferior. Journal of Nutrition Dietetics 1993;6:355–371.
5. Davis, EA. Functionality of sugars. American Journal of Clinical Nutrition 1995.
6. Bright-See E, Jazmaji V. Estimation of amount of dietary starch available to different populations. Canadian Journal of Physiology and Pharmacology 1991;69:56–59.
7. Sigman-Grant M, Stanton J, Keast DR, Gibney M. Consumption of sugars in the United States and in the European Union. American Journal of Clinical Nutrition 1995.
8. Baghurst KI, Record SJ, Syrette JA, Crawford DA, Baghurst PA. Intakes and sources of a range of dietary sugars in various Australian populations. Medical Journal of Australia 1989;151:512–518.

9. Glinnsmann WH, Irausquin H, Park Y. Evaluation of health aspects of sugars contained in carbohydrate sweeteners. Report of the Sugars Task Force 1986. Washington: US Food and Drug Administration, 1986.

10. Department of Health and Community Services. Dietary sugars and human disease. Report of the panel on dietary sugars. London: Her Majesty's Stationery Office, 1989; vol Report on health and social subjects no. 37.).

11. Sokoloff L, Fitzgerald G, Kaufman EE. Cerebral nutrition and energy metabolism. In: Nutrition and the brain. New York: Raven Press, 1977:87–139. vol 1).

12. Frienkel N. Of pregnancy and progeny. Diabetes 1980;29:1023–1034.

13. Gray GM. Starch digestion and absorption in nonruminants. Journal of Nutrition 1992;122:172–177.

14. Brand JC, Nicholson PL, Thorburn AW, Truswell AS. Food processing and the glycemic index. American Journal of Clinical Nutrition 1985;42:1192–1196.

15. Ross SW, Brand JC, Thorburn AW, Truswell AS. Glycaemic index of processed wheat products. American Journal of Chemical Nutrition 1987;46:631–635.

16. Behall KM, Schofield DJ, Canary J. Effect of starch structure on glucose and insulin responses in adults. American Journal of Clinical Nutrition 1988;47:428–432.

17. Heaton KW, Marcus SN, Emmett PM, Bolton CH. Particle size of wheat, maize, and oat test meals: effects on

plasma glucose and insulin responses and on the rate of starch digestion in vitro. American Journal of Clinical Nutrition 1988;47:675–682.

18. Scrimshaw NS, Murray EB. The acceptability of milk and milk products in populations with a high prevalence of lactose intolerance. American Journal of Clinical Nutrition 1988;48 (suppl):1083–1159.

19. Englyst HN, Kingman SM, Cummings JH. Classification and measurement of nutritionally important starch fractions. European Journal of Clinical Nutrition 1992;46(suppl2):S33–S50.

20. Flourie B, Leblond A, Florent C, Rautureau M, Biscall A, Rambaud J-C. Starch malabsorption and breath gas excretion in healthy humans consuming low- and high-starch diets. Gastroenterology 1988;95:356–363.

21. Thornton JR, Dryden A, Kelleher J, Losowsky MS. Dig Dis Sci 1987;32:1088–1091.

22. Truswell AS, Seach JM, Thorburn AW. Incomplete absorption of pure fructose in healthy subjects and the facilitating effect of glucose. American Journal of Clinical Nutrition 1988;48:1424–1430.

23. Yki-Jarvinen H. Action of insulin on glucose metabolism in vivo. Bailliere's Clinical Endocrinology and Metabolism 1993;7:903–927.

24. Jenkins DJA, Wolever TM, Jenkins AL. Starchy foods and glycemic index. Diabetes Care 1988;11:149–159.

25. Brand-Miller, J, Pang E, Broomhead L. The glycaemic index of foods containing sugars: comparison of foods with naturally-occurring vs added sugars. British Journal of Nutrition 1995;73:613–623.

26. Jenkins DJA, Wolever TMS, Taylor R. Glycaemic index of foods: a physiological basis for carbohydrate exchange. American Journal of Clinical Nutrition 1981;34:362–366.

27. Fontvieille AM, Acosta M, Rizkalla SW. A moderate switch from high to low glycemic-index foods for 3 weeks improves metabolic control of Type 1 (IDDM) diabetic subjects. Diabetes Nutrition and Metabolism 1988;1:139–143.

28. Brand-Miller J. The importance of glycemic index in diabetes. American Journal of Clinical Nutrition 1994;59(suppl):747S–752S.

29. Thomas DE, Brotherhood JR, Brand JC. Carbohydrate feeding before exercise: effect of glycemic index. International Journal of Sports Nutrition 1991;12:180–186.

30. Holt S, Brand J, Soveny C, Hansky J. Relationship of satiety to postprandial glycemic, insulin and cholecystokinin responses. Appetite 1992;18:129–141.

31. Lyons PM, Truswell AS. Serotonin precursor influenced by type of carbohydrate meal in healthy adults. American Journal of Clinical Nutrition 1988;47:433–43.

32. Jequier E. Carbohydrates as a source of energy. American

Journal of Clinical Nutrition 1994;59(suppl):682S–685S.

33. Acheson KJ, Schulz Y, Bessard T, Flatt JP, Jequier E. Carbohydrate metabolism and de novo lipogenesis in human obesity. American Journal of Clinical Nutrition 1987;45:78–85.

34. Delarue J, S. N, Pachiaudi C, Beylot M, Lamisse F, Riou JP. The contribution of naturally labelled 13C fructose to glucose appearance in humans. Diabetologia 1993;36:338–345.

35. Brown SS, Forest Jan, Roscoe P. Associated trial of fructose in the treatment of acute alcoholic intoxication. Lancet 1972;2:898–899.

36. Kalchar HM. Science 1965;150:305–313.

37. Navia JM. Carbohydrates and dental health. American Journal of Clinical Nutrition 1994;59(suppl):719S–727S.

38. Truswell AS. Sugar and health: a review. Food Technology in Australia 1987;39:134–140.

39. Peterson DB, Lambert J, Gerring S, et al. Sugar in the diet of diabetic patients – just another carbohydrate? Diabetologia 1986;29:216–220.

40. Colagiuri S, Miller JJ, Edwards RA. Metabolic effects of adding sugar and aspartame to the diet of subjects with noninsulin-dependent diabetes mellitus. American Journal of Clinical Nutrition 1989;50:474–478.

41. Sheppard L, Kristal AR, Kushi LH. Weight loss in women participating in a randomized trial of low-fat diets.

American Journal of Clinical Nutrition 1991;54:821–828.

42. Ravussin E, Schultz Y, Acheson KJ, Dusmet M, Bourquin L, Jequier E. Short-term, mixed diet overfeeding in man: no evidence for 'luxusconsumption'. American Journal of Physiology 1985;249:E470–E477.

43. Lissner, L, Livitsky DA. Dietary fat and the regulation of energy intake in human subjects. American Journal of Clinical Nutrition 1987;46:886–892.

44. Green SM, Burley VJ, Blundell JE. Effect of fat- and sugar-containing food on the size of eating episodes and energy intake in lean males: potential for causing overconsumption. European Journal of Clinical Nutrition 1994;48:547–555.

45. Cotton, JR, Burley VJ, Weststrate JA, Blundell JE. Dietary fat and appetite: similarities and differences in the satiating effect of meals supplemented with either fat or carbohydrate. Journal of Human Nutrition and Dietetics 1994;7:11–24.

46. Acheson KJ, Schutz Y, Bessard T, Amantharaman K, Flatt JP, Jequier E. Glycogen storage capacity and de novo lipogenesis during massive carbohydrate overfeeding in man. American Journal of Clinical Nutrition 1988;48:240–247.

47. Truswell AS. Food carbohydrates and plasma lipids – an update. American Journal of Clinical Nutrition 1994;59(suppl):710S–718S.

48. Garg A, Scott M, Unger RH. Comparison of effects of high and low carbohydrate diets on plasma lipoproteins and insulin sensitivity in patients with mild NIDDM. Diabetes 1992;41:1278–1285.

49. Nutrition AAoPCo. The practical significance of lactose intolerance in children. Pediatrics 1978;62:240–245.

50. Kolars JC, Levitt MD, Aouji M, Savaiano DA. Yogurt – an autodigesting source of lactose. New England Journal of Medicine 1984;310:1–3.

51. Trowell HC, Burkitt DP. Refined carbohydrates in health and disease. London: Academic Press, 1975.

52. Prosky L, Asp NG, Schweizer TF et al. Determination of insoluble, soluble and total dietary fibre in foods and food products: interlaboratory study. Journal of Association Official Analytical Chemists 1988;71:1017–1023.

53. Englyst H, Cummings J. Improved method for measurement of dietary fibre as non-starch polysaccharides in plant food. Journal of Association of Official Analytical Chemists 1988;71:808–814.

54. Cummings JH. Fermentation in the human large intestine: evidence and implications for health. Lancet 1983;1:1206–1209.

55. Cummings JH. Carbohydrate fermentation in the human large bowel: its control and consequences. In: Malnutrition in chronic diet-associated infantile diarrhoea. 1989:305–331.

56. British Nutrition Foundation. Complex carbohydrates in food. The report of the British Nutrition Foundation's Task Force. London: Chapman and Hall, 1990.

57. Vinik AI, Jenkins DJA. Dietary fibre in management of diabetes. Diabetes Care 1988;11:160–73.

58. Haber GB, Heaton KW, Murphy D, Burroughs L. Depletion and disruption of dietary fibre: effect on satiety, plasma glucose and serum insulin. Lancet 1977;2:6796–82.

59. Riccardi G, Rivellese AA. Can diabetes mellitus be prevented by diet? Diabet Nutr Metab 1989;2:259–262.

60. Mann J. Diabetic dietary prescriptions. Br Med J 1989;298:1535–1536.

61. Reavan GM. Dietary therapy in non-insulin-dependent diabetes mellitus. New Engl J Med 1988;319:862–864.

62. Truswell AS, Kay RM. Absence of effect of bran on blood lipids. Lancet 1975;1:922–923.

63. Anderson JW, Story L, Sieling B, Che WL, Petro MS, Story J. Hypocholesterolaemic effects of high fibre diets rich in water-soluble plant fibres. J Can Diet Assoc 1984;451:140–149.

64. Jenkins DJA. Carbohydrates (B) Dietary fibre. In: Shils ME, Young VR, ed. Modern nutrition in health and disease. Philadelphia: Lea & Febiger, 1988.

65. Heaton KW, Manning AP, Hartog M. Lack of effect on blood lipids and calcium concentrations of young men on

changing from white to wholemeal bread. Br J Nutr
1986;35:55–60.

66. Willet W. The search for the causes of breast and colon
    cancer. Nature 1989;338:389–394.

67. McKeown-Eyssen GE, Bright-See E. Dietary factors in
    colon cancer: international relationships. Nutrition and
    Cancer 1984;6:160–170.

68. Cummings JH. Constipation, dietary fibre and control of
    large bowel function. Postgraduate Medical Journal
    1984;60:811–819.

69. James WPT. Dietary fibre and mineral metabolism. 3. In:
    Spiller GA, Kay RM, ed. Medical aspects of dietary fibre.
    New York: Plenum Press, 1980:239.

ABOUT THE AUTHORS

Kaye Foster-Powell, an accredited practising dietitian-nutritionist, has extensive experience in diabetes management and has researched practical applications of the glycaemic index. She is the senior dietitian at Wentworth Area Diabetes Service and conducts a private practice in the Blue Mountains, NSW.

Jennie Brand-Miller is Associate Professor of Human Nutrition in the Human Nutrition Unit at the University of Sydney. She is a world authority on the glycaemic index of foods and its applications to health.

Dr Anthony Leeds is Senior Lecturer in the Department of Nutrition & Dietetics at King's College London. He graduated in medicine from the Middlesex Hospital Medical School, London, UK in 1971. He conducts research on carbohydrate and dietary fibre in relation to heart disease, obesity and diabetes and continues part-time medical practice. He chairs the research ethics committee of King's College London, is a member of the Society of Authors, and in 1999 was elected a Fellow of the Institute of Biology.